Shopping Addiction

A simple solution guide to begin your journey towards breaking your shopping addiction and compulsive buying

By. Nadhia Korsacova

Introduction

I want to thank you and congratulate you for downloading the book, 'Shopping Addiction Reformation."
Do you always find yourself buying more than you need no matter how much you promise yourself that this time would be different? Have you gotten yourself into financial troubles because of your overspending? Do you often feel unsatisfied and empty after a spending spree? If this is you, then you may be addicted to shopping.

Like any other form of addiction, shopping addiction is a habit that usually develops over time either as a way to cope with something or as the only way you know how to reward yourself. That said, compulsive buying never helps but rather only makes things worse.

The good news is that there is hope; you can actually overcome shopping addiction and start enjoying shopping for things you actually need and not buying compulsively. This book outlines the steps you need to take now to change your life and free yourself from the chains of shopping addiction.

© **Copyright 2018 - All rights reserved.**

This document is geared towards providing exact and reliable information in regards to the topic and issue covered. The publication is sold with the idea that the publisher is not required to render accounting, officially permitted, or otherwise, qualified services. If advice is necessary, legal or professional, a practiced individual in the profession should be ordered.

- From a Declaration of Principles which was accepted and approved equally by a Committee of the American Bar Association and a Committee of Publishers and Associations.

In no way is it legal to reproduce, duplicate, or transmit any part of this document in either electronic means or in printed format. Recording of this publication is strictly prohibited and any storage of this document is not allowed unless with written permission from the publisher. All rights reserved.

The information provided herein is stated to be truthful and consistent, in that any liability, in terms of inattention or otherwise, by any usage or abuse of any policies, processes, or directions contained within is the solitary and utter responsibility of the recipient reader. Under no circumstances will any legal responsibility or blame be held against the publisher for any reparation, damages, or monetary loss due to the information herein, either directly or indirectly.

Respective authors own all copyrights not held by the publisher.

The information herein is offered for informational purposes solely, and is universal as so. The presentation of the information is without contract or any type of guarantee assurance.

The trademarks that are used are without any consent, and the publication of the trademark is without permission or backing by the trademark owner. All trademarks and brands within this book are for clarifying purposes only and are the owned by the owners themselves, not affiliated with this document.

Shopping Addiction Reformation

Table of Contents

Introduction
Chapter 1: Shopping Addiction - The 5 Stages Of Compulsive Shopping
Chapter 2: Are You Addicted To Shopping?
Chapter 3: How Media & Advertising Affects And Manipulates Your Shopping Habits
Chapter 4: How To Overcome Shopping Addiction
Chapter 5: Battling Your Triggers And Finding Healthier Alternatives To Shopping
Conclusion

Chapter 1: Shopping Addiction - The 5 Stages Of Compulsive Shopping

Also known as **oniomania** or **compulsive buying disorder** (CBD), shopping addiction is simply the urge to spend money in an excessive, inappropriate manner that is out of control. Like any other type of addiction, when you are addicted to shopping, you usually lack control over your spending impulses.

Compulsive shopping is a process that usually follows 5 phases according to researchers who published a review of CDB in the journal of World Psychiatry.

1. **Anticipation**

At this stage, you may see, hear or read advertisements on the mainstream media or social media. Your mind then becomes preoccupied with thoughts and cravings of shopping. You become excited about the possibility of purchasing something or everything.

2. **Preparation**

You then start to plan how you are going to go shopping. This is the stage where you begin to think about how you will dress up, make the funds available and think about what stores you will visit. Sense of euphoria begins to heighten from this stage.

3. **Shopping**

This is the main act and is extremely pleasurable. Usually this sense of euphoria comes with fulfillment of completing your mission. Some researchers even noted that some shoppers experience a sexual feeling as they shop.

4. **Spending**

This is the time when you have to pay for the goods or services immediately or through a monthly bill. Paying with cash is more painful than paying with a credit card. Credit cards separate the pain of paying from the pleasure of buying. Whenever you use a credit card, you are seduced into thinking only about the positive aspects of a purchase.

5. **Remorse**

From here you begin to feel let down, remorseful, ashamed, depressed, guilty among other negative feelings and thoughts. This phase typically takes a lot of emotional energy and time. At times, you may even decide to hide the items, discard them, sell them, give them away or return them to the store. The result is a vicious cycle in which that negative feeling fuels you to obtain another 'shopping fix'

With that basic understanding of shopping addiction and the different phases, let us now move on to finding out if you are actually a shopping addict.

Chapter 2: Are You Addicted To Shopping

Before we move on to the steps you need to take now to deal with the addiction, let us first evaluate your behavior to be sure that you are actually addicted to shopping.

When you suffer from a shopping addiction:

You experience a rush of excitement when you purchase

If you are a shopping addict, you are likely to experience an adrenaline rush or a 'shopper's high' after purchasing something. This euphoric feeling does not come from owning what you just bought, but from the act of buying it. The brain releases dopamine and endorphins in waves when you see a desirable item worth buying. The triggering of chemical reactions in the brain generates a real high. Naturally, you want to experience this high over and over again. It is this repeated behavior, which eventually spirals into an addiction.

You feel remorseful after shopping

When buying, you are so often caught up in the thrill of the moment but remorse and regret usually set in when you receive your credit card statement via email or once you get home. Sometimes you feel remorseful if the shopping spree contradicts with promises you made to a loved one or yourself. Mostly though, the guilt arises from the irresponsible purchases that your perceive as indulges. The consequence is a vicious cycle. This negative feeling of guilt fuels you to seek another 'fix' by purchasing some more items.

You make frequent impulse purchases

Purchasing things you never planned to buy or do not need in the first place is a strong indicator of shopping addiction. This means that you purchase items that you never or almost never use. In other words, you only buy for no other reason other than to spend money; and experience that rush of excitement when paying at the counter. Once you are satisfied with the urge of purchasing, you completely lose interest in the item you bought. For this reason, you'll usually find tagged clothes and plenty of unopened boxes in your home. With time, you become a hoarder.

You shop as a reaction to anger, stress, fear or disappointment

In the same way, an alcohol addict will crave for alcohol when faced with a challenging situation; you will rush to the shopping mall to help ease stressful thoughts or the feelings of anxiety. You will tend to buy things to help you fill an emotional void caused by either loneliness or lack of self-confidence; the reason being that making a new purchase releases the feel good chemicals that make you feel relieved. However, this decrease in the negative emotions is short lived and is quickly replaced with guilt and anxiety.

You lie about the extensive shopping habits to family and friends

You may not admit it to other people but deep down you know that your compulsive spending is problematic. For this reason, you will go to great lengths to hide your behavior from people who care about you to avoid worrying them. Another reason why you will want to keep your spending secret is that it intensifies your shopping thrill. Therefore, if you notice that you have deceptive behaviors such as hiding shopping bags in the closet or car or deleting your browser history after shopping online then you may be addicted to shopping.

You become anxious when you go for an extended period without shopping

As a shopping addict, you usually report feeling 'out of sorts' if you haven't had your regular shopping fix. If that is the case, you will usually resort to shopping online if you are unable to pull away from your day-to-day activities.

Now that you are aware of the symptoms of the problem, here is a little exercise that I want you to do.

Exercise

For a few days, observe your behavior and attitude to better understand your problem and diagnose it properly. If you can, ask a trustworthy friend to be your accountability and support and ask him/her to observe you. Look for any of these signs to easily identify your problem. Make sure to write it down in a journal and go through it a few times to acknowledge if you may need help and have a problem that is affecting your life.

Chapter 3: How Media & Advertising Affects And Manipulates Your Shopping Habits

You may probably be wondering how you got yourself here in the first place. Well, the truth is that you are not the only one to blame for your addiction; the media has also played a part. Understanding how the media has contributed to your addiction and how adverts affect you is crucial to ensure that once you overcome shopping addiction, you don't relapse because you will be better informed.

How Adverts Can Manipulate You

The thing is, advertising is important because it helps you become aware of an useful product you didn't know about, it helps create demand for products and above all, it also enables you to choose from a number of products already in the market. While adverts aren't bad, most of them are manipulative.

Ads nowadays are more complex and usually involve cinematic messages whose intention is to make significant memories of a product. The memories are created because the ad achieves its aim of making you come up with an emotional response, which can have a great effect on how you think and the kind of choices you make.

There are different kinds of ads but they all have one thing in common; they all bar you from thinking so that you may make purchasing choices based on an emotional response.

Whenever there is competition between or among companies or service providers that offer the same service, the ads you see will be more descriptive so as to set one product or service apart from the other. For instance, a fast food company may be selling reasonably tasty but unhealthy hot dogs. However, they will still convince you to choose theirs over another. Why? Because they say so. To help you understand this better consider the following study conducted by Ellen Langer and her team to provide a very interesting demonstration regarding how easy it can be to persuade people to take action.

In the research, an undercover experimenter approached a group of students in a library and requested to jump ahead of them in the photocopying queue to make himself some copies. At times, the experimenter would justify his request by saying, "May I kindly use the Xerox machine because I am in a hurry?"

Sometimes he never offered any explanation at all. Surprisingly, most of the students were not willing to grant his request when he did not make an effort to justify it. The funny thing is that the justification never had to give the students a good reason; it only needed to seem like one. Thus, the students readily complied to the experimenter's favor when he gave them a seemingly 'placebo' explanation that essentially had no content: "May I kindly use the Xerox machine because I am in a hurry?" Apparently, the experimenter only had to 'decorate' his request with the 'Xerox' word and it proved just enough to persuade them.

That said, advertisers would seek to confuse you with pseudoscience. They can trick you by either use of vaguely cited research and scientific-sounding jargon so that you may think that their product is very credible.

So what do you do to avoid this? When you come right down to it, you have to be prepared to think and be alert. Most of the times you are not often prepared to think when perusing through a magazine or when watching TV. This means that you will readily accept any suggestion that is presented in front of you, and in view of the fact that you are just passive, you will never realize that it has happened.

Think about what the ad is talking about. Don't be subconscious when watching a commercial. Try to determine if there is any negative aspect about the product being advertised that definitely is not being brought to your attention. If you keep your brain active when viewing an ad, you will be in a better position to make sound decisions.

Emotional Responses to Ads

If you have ever bought something not because it is functional but because it appeals to you, then you made an emotional choice fuelled by your desires instead of thinking logically about it.

Being emotional isn't necessarily a bad thing. However, if you do not make an effort to balance logic and emotion, you will not usually make the right decisions. Ads that appeal to your emotions take advantage of this phenomenon. Such ads get you to purchase an item, but not to buy the item and be happy with it.

If you notice that you are emotionally responsive to advertisements, you have to be cautious about the choices you are going to make regarding the item on sale. The good thing is that the arousal of emotions wears off with time, which means that you can avoid falling prey to spending on unnecessary stuff that will make you feel terrible afterwards.

First, whenever you are thinking about purchasing a product, you need to determine whether your motivation is extrinsic or intrinsic. If you are an extrinsically motivated person, you focus on appearance, financial gain and social popularity. Basically, you seek acceptance by someone or something outside yourself.

On the other hand, if you are intrinsically motivated, your behavior will be driven by natural rewards. In other words, you do something because you honestly love to do it or because you find it interesting.

That said you would need to avoid buying anything you believe you want if your motivation is extrinsic. The reason is because your desire will usually be great and chances are you will be addicted to spending.

To help you overcome this, the best thing to do is to implement an enforced holding pattern on how you spend. Basically, the idea is to not buy whatever you think you need for two days. You may ask a friend you trust to help you with this one. Let him/her hold onto your credit card for that period and make them the gatekeeper to what you buy.

How Social Media Influences Your Shopping Addiction

Social media began as a platform for people to share photos of their family and friends and stay in touch with one another. However, it has now evolved into an impactful platform for businesses. According to Sprout Social, more than 74% of people make purchasing decisions with the help of social media.

A study conducted by business school researchers reveals that social media can really influence the amount of money you spend when shopping to a point where you can't control yourself. If you notice that you are spending too much money on shopping, there are some factors you need to consider as far as social media is concerned.

The internet is an essential part of life today. Social media is a regular fixture in particular. It enables you to connect with other people and these connections influence your life in one way or another. As you make these connections, you build up trust with the people you are connected to. For instance, you are more likely to believe in what your peers and role models on social media say and recommend especially if they are your friends or family. One study that was conducted by Market World Research shows that 25% of internet users trust what their family and friends post on social media, 26% trust what is written on their blog posts, 20% trust tweets. This is in contrast to 5% who trust tweets of strangers and 7% who trust posts and blogs of strangers.

Apart from family and friends, there are also social influencers who affect your buying behavior. These people who have a significant following on social media. These influencers have a large audience and for that reason, they are targeted by businesses to help promote their products and services.

Nevertheless, irrespective of whether some of the posts by social influencers are sponsored by businesses or not, whatever they post seems to have an effect on consumer purchasing decisions. Basically, they contribute to the bandwagon effect.

For instance, if a social influencer posts on Facebook about his/her newly acquired pair of shoes and talks about how affordable and comfortable they are, the audience will be interested to learn more about the shoes.

When connections are made and trust is built, you as the consumer will more likely spend based on what other people you are connected to post on the internet. That said, the internet and social media exposes you to services and items that you may actually not have been aware of. While internet, social media and different marketing media do influence us positively too, they are largely to be blamed for compelling us to become addicted to shopping. Fortunately, this problem can be treated effectively and if you are committed to overcoming shopping addiction for good, move on to the next chapter to find out the first step to do so.

Chapter 4: How To Overcome Shopping Addiction

From this point forward, the book will focus on steps you need to take to overcome shopping addiction.

Step 1 - Set A Dedicated Intention And Commitment

The first step to overcome any addiction whether drug, alcohol or shopping, is to set an unwavering commitment to do so. Unless you are committed to a goal, you will not work dedicatedly to achieve it and are quite likely to quit its pursuit especially in times when you experience an incredibly strong urge to succumb to your temptations. The same applies to compulsive shopping. If you don't completely dedicate yourself to the mission of breaking this unhealthy addiction, you are quite likely to browse through e-stores or even visit the real stores after some time and end up making an actual purchase.

Here's how you can commit yourself to the goal:

Visualize How Your Addiction has Influenced Your Life

A good technique to become committed to a goal is to focus on why you wish to change. You need to back every goal that you set with some compelling reasons why you wish to achieve it. When you don't have compelling reasons why you must work on a goal, you are quite likely to go off the track the minute the going gets tough and when you feel you can no longer put up with the tough goal.

As opposed to this, when you are clear on why you want to actualize a goal, you revisit the reasons every time your motivation levels drop low. Those reasons fuel your commitment and make you focus on your end goal constantly so instead of giving up on it, you power through and make sure to follow through with it until the very end.

Think of How Compulsive Shopping Impacts You Negatively

To find out why overcoming your shopping addiction is essential for you, visualize how it affects your life and how your life will change for the better once you break the addiction for good.

Sit somewhere quiet and peaceful and carry your journal along. Sit comfortably in any pose that suits you well and close your eyes. Start by thinking of a happy memory that helps you unwind such as the time you went on a vacation with your family or the time you held your baby in your arms for the first time, or anything else that puts a smile on your face and helps you feel calm.

When you feel better, think of how your shopping addiction has influenced your life negatively. Think about how you fall short of saving money every time you plan to do it because you just cannot stop spending it on clothes or shoes or gadgets. Think of how it has heightened your stress and makes you edgy all the time. Ponder on how it makes you think incessantly about buying more stuff only and never lets your mind rest making you feel chaotic all the time. Focus on how your shopping addiction has adversely affected your time management skills and how you cannot find the time to complete your tasks on time ever. Think about how you keep delaying your assignments because you stay hooked online on e-stores for hours and hours. Ponder on all the money you owe to your friends and family because you could not resist the urge to buy new chairs, rugs and wall art for your house. Go through all these factors and all the other reasons why your addiction has made your life difficult, miserable and uncomfortable.

A wise move would be to write down all these findings and go through them a few times to imbed all these things in your mind. When you keep thinking of how your addiction has increased your suffering, you feel more motivated from within to work on breaking it. These are also the reasons why you MUST work on overcoming this bad habit and push you towards fulfilling your commitment.

Next, you need to strengthen this newfound motivation by focusing on how your life will change for the better once you have broken this addiction for good.

Think of How Overcoming Compulsive Shopping will Improve Your Life

Close your eyes or keep them open if you want and think deeply about how overcoming this compulsive shopping behavior will add positivity, value and meaning to your life. Think of how relaxed and free you will feel emotionally when you are not governed by your addiction. Think of the emotional stability that you will get to enjoy once you have completely controlled your addiction. Think of how you will slowly be able to save money when you do not spend all your hard-earned income on making unnecessary and impulse purchases.

Focus on how you will save your house of all the unnecessary clutter and make only meaningful purchases. Ponder on how you will be able to save more time and use it wisely instead of wasting away hours moving from one store to another or gazing at magazines, both real and online planning your next shopping spree. Think about how you will be able to work on tasks that are more meaningful with greater focus and complete them on time instead of procrastinating until the end and greatly affecting your productivity.

Also, think of how you will spare yourself of the undue stress and tension you have brought onto yourself primarily because you cannot keep yourself from making more purchases.

Think of how your focus will improve and how you will slowly be able to concentrate on your goal and pursue your ambitions to live a more meaningful life.

Ponder on how you will slowly turn into a happier, calm soul from a grumpy, agitated one because you don't feel compelled to do something you don't genuinely want to do.

Think of how you will start spending your money on meaningful purchases and ideas and use them positively instead of spending your money on things you think you need, but don't really require to purchase.

Focus on how your relationships will improve because you will be able to spend more time with the people you love now that you no longer spend hours window-shopping.

Like before, write down all these reasons as well, so you can go through the account and drive energy from it to further fuel your commitment towards your goal. Speak them out loudly as it makes you focus better on them and makes them imbed in your mind, which then positively influences your actions. Your next task is to set a real intention and create a goal based on your commitment.

Formulate Your Commitment and Goal

Now that you are well aware of your problem and the need to address it, document your commitment to solidify it. Take out your journal and write down exactly what you wish to do and turn it into a real time goal.

For instance, if you wish to overcome your shopping addiction, think of why you wish to do that by going over the accounts you created earlier again and think of a reasonable timeframe you would require to work on this very goal. You can say, 'I am addicted to compulsive shopping, but I am committed to breaking this addiction for good to live a more peaceful and meaningful life."

When you write it down, speak it loudly, slowly and confidently a few times to plough its seeds in your subconscious mind. When you say something repeatedly with deep conviction, you divert your subconscious mind's focus to it.

There is a filter in your brain known as the 'Reticular Activating System' (RAS) that filters out unnecessary information that you pick to prevent information overload. Whatever thing you focus on and have repeatedly said or done becomes the center of your focus and is considered as important by the RAS. When your RAS deems something as significant, it directs your attention towards it making you concentrate more on it. As you focus more on something, you create more thoughts based on it. Your thoughts travel out in the universe and draw towards them other thoughts of similar vibrations. With those thoughts, come all the experiences tied to them as well so if you think positively and focus on achieving your goal, you will create more thoughts in that direction and attract similar thoughts towards yourself and increase your chances of fulfilling your goal.

Therefore, when you write down your commitment, speak it loudly and clearly about 15 to 20 times to fix your focus on it and rewire your brain to think in that direction. Next, you need to create a SMART goal based on your commitment to make it easier for you to work on it.

SMART Goal

SMART is a tool to create meaningful, specific and clear goals that you easily understand and can work on effectively. With a SMART goal, you become better aware of the goal you need to work on, when it is due, how realistic and attainable it is, and how you can measure your performance related to it. SMART stands for specific, measurable, attainable, realistic and time-tagged.

Here is how to set a meaningful SMART goal for yourself: Specific: A specific goal is one that clearly states what you are trying to achieve. Trying to live a healthy life isn't as clear as trying to live a healthy life by overcoming internet addiction. With a specific goal, you know exactly what you are chasing and don't feel confused. Thus, when you decide to break your shopping addiction, tie it to why you want to do it and the effect it will bring in your life. For instance, your specific goal could be, 'I am committed to overcome my shopping addiction so that I can have better control over my finances and to live a happier more empowered life.'

Measurable: Measurable goals are those that you can easily keep track of and measure the performance of. This helps you keep track of your milestones and be aware of how well or poorly you have been working towards your goals. Therefore, if you are trying to overcome the urge to shop obsessively, think about the tool you will use to measure how you have been working on that commitment. Will you keep a check on your expenses and use an increase or decrease in them to analyze your performance or will you analyze your savings and look for an increase in it because that would mean you are spending less on buying unnecessary stuff. Identify a system to measure your performance; one that suits your style and stick to it to assess how smoothly you work towards the fulfillment of your goal.

Attainable: An attainable goal is one that you can achieve using all the resources you have available to you. For example, if you are trying to overcome your shopping addiction, think of all the resources that you have and then plan how to utilize them to achieve your goal. It is important to set attainable goals so that you do not put off your goal for a time when you have everything available at your disposal and can get started to achieve it right now making use of whatever resources you have.

Realistic: A realistic goal is one that is not far-fetched and feels realistically achievable and possible. For instance, breaking an addiction that you have been having for 2 years cannot be easily broken in a month so a realistic goal in this case would be to give yourself at least 8 to 10 months to overcome the addiction. Think of how long you have been addicted and then set a realistic goal accordingly.

Time-tagged: A time-tagged goal is one with a deadline attached to it. Having a deadline with your goal is important so that you do not keep procrastinating and work on it right away because you know when it is due. Take into account, the pace at which you work, how strong your addiction is and the environment you work in before setting a deadline. If you work at a moderate pace, spend thousands of dollars on shopping every week and find it very hard to control your urges even for a few hours, you need anywhere from 6 to 12 months to completely rid yourself of this addiction. However, if you have been addicted to shopping for a few months only and spend a few hundred dollars on shopping stuff once every month, but you know those are all meaningless and unimportant purchases, you can break off your addiction in 1 to 3 months.

Once you have set a SMART goal, analyze it a few times to ensure you have set the right requirements and feel good about your goal. Your next task is to dig deeper into the issue and search for any underlying causes and reasons that may be triggering your addiction and fueling it as well.

Step 2 - Digging Deeper Into The Problem

Any addiction is mostly rooted in some other problem that exacerbates over time and makes you resort to a certain tempting behavior or practice to assuage your feelings. You may be going through a traumatic experience in your life and cannot handle the stress alone so you turn to smoking to relieve it. Similarly, it is quite likely that there is some other problem behind your compulsive buying behavior that is pushing you to engage in it.

To overcome your addiction, it is imperative to delve deeper into the problem and identify the root cause. Let us see how you can do that successfully:

Ponder on the Root Cause

Think about your life and the way you feel right now and pour down those feelings in your journal. If writing is not your thing and it weighs you down, speak about your feelings and record them.

If you are not happy with the state of your life right now and if there is something wrong going on that is constantly stressing you out, it is likely that you resort to shopping to feel good. Since this does the trick, you keep engaging in that behavior repeatedly to enjoy that happy feeling over and over again.

Try to pinpoint the troubles you are going through and better understand your emotions that make you feel uneasy and then somehow encourage you to shop.

Also, think of the first time you shopped like crazy and try to figure out why you did so. Maybe you hadn't shopped in a while because you never had enough money and that one time, you had sort of hit a jackpot or had extra money to splurge on yourself and so you did. You felt great spending without thinking much and the feelings of joy and power you enjoyed were strong enough to make you want to engage in other shopping sprees shortly after. Maybe that was why you soon became addicted to shopping and haven't been able to break that bad habit until now. Your underlying cause fueling your addiction can be different, but make sure to think about it so you can move towards recovering it easily.

According to John A. Roberts, who has a PhD, and is the author of the book 'Too Much of a Good Thing' and is a professor of marketing at the Baylor University, he believes that compulsive shopping is actually a means to fill some sort of emptiness people are experiencing in one or more aspects of their lives. This could include unhealthy relationships, bad job, depression etc. If someone isn't too happy with his spouse, he may find it soothing to turn to Amazon to feel better.

As you work on identifying the root cause, focus on understanding your triggers too because sometimes, there isn't one strong reason that makes you lean towards an addiction, but a series of different events that slowly make you inculcate a certain habit you aren't too proud of.

Pay Attention to Your Triggers

Spend some time analyzing what triggers you to shop. Every habit, be it a good, bad or neutral one follows a certain cycle. It starts with a trigger or a reminder, which can be an act, an object, a certain time of the day, a feeling, a thought or a certain person that reminds you of a certain practice.

This then leads to the routine, which refers to how you engage in that habit followed by rewards. Rewards refer to all the benefits you derive out of that practice that make you want to engage in the practice repeatedly. I'll share an example with you to better help you understand this cycle. Each time you feel bored, you open your laptop or pick up your Smart phone and head straight to Amazon.com to browse through different products. Boredom here is the feeling that triggered your compulsive shopping behavior. So, you start browsing through the site and come across different products of which you select 5 and place the order. This is the routine. Once the order had been placed and even throughout the process of browsing, selecting and placing the order, you feel excited, happy and less bored than before. These emotions are your rewards that you enjoy after engaging in the respective activity, and of course, the fact that you will have more of the things you like in a few days. It is such feelings that make you stick to the bad habit for good.

To break this vicious cycle of surrendering to your addiction repeatedly, you need to take a moment to identify your triggers. Be aware of your different emotions, feelings and thoughts along with the different incidents and experiences you go through and see how each one of them shapes you and turns you towards your addiction. For that, you will have to inculcate mindfulness in you.

Become Mindful to Better Understand Yourself and Your Triggers

Mindfulness refers to living in the moment in a nonjudgmental, peaceful and accepting manner so that you accept everything as it comes to you and are aware of every moment that passes by.

This moment by moment awareness and the acceptance of everything that comes your way makes you more conscious of what happens to you without putting any sort of negative labels on your feelings.

Therefore, if you are mindful, you won't judge yourself for feeling envious of the gorgeous dress your friend is wearing and looking it up online to buy the same for yourself, but would accept your envy as a very normal emotion that you are feeling and one that can be addressed in another way.

This calms you down and helps you think clearly. Otherwise, you would have just given in to your temptations and feelings right away without thinking twice about how that affects you and would have just made a meaningless purchase or two and only increased your burden.

Also, mindfulness helps you better identify the different series of events that trigger your addiction and make you engage in it. If you cannot think clearly and focus on one thought at a time, you are likely to take all the thoughts as a whole and become overwhelmed by them, and eventually resort to binge shopping.

When you have the ability to pause, take some time-out and focus on one thought at a time, you can analyze its implications and address it before it takes an evil turn. Hence, to overcome your shopping addiction successfully, you need to slowly train yourself to become more mindful. While there are many ways to do that, a simple and super-effective technique is to practice mindfulness-breathing meditation for just 5 minutes daily.

Mindfulness Breathing Meditation

You can practice this simple exercise at any hour of the day and even anywhere to bring a sense of calmness, focus and awareness and really live in the moment. Here's how you can practice it.

- Sit comfortably in a quiet room or even a noisy room if you can maintain focus in it. Set a timer for 5 minutes and if that seems quite long, set it for 2 minutes.

- Close your eyes and think of anything that calms you down for a few seconds.

- As you feel better, very gently, bring your attention to your breath and pay attention to how you inhale and exhale. Inhale through your nose, observe your breath flowing in and extending to your belly, exhale through your mouth, and focus on how expelling the air makes you feel.

- Keep watching your breath in this manner and whenever you feel even the least bit distracted, remind yourself of the practice at hand and slowly bring back your awareness to your breath. Remember to be calm with yourself and don't let agitation take over. You can count your breath too to stay more focused on it.

- Keep observing your breath for 2 to 5 minutes and when your timer beeps, gently bring back your attention to the real world and slowly open your eyes.

- Enjoy the feeling of calmness you instilled inside you and relish it for a few minutes. You will find yourself feeling clearer and fresher than before.

Practice this exercise daily and if you can, perform it twice every day, once in the morning and once at night. If you do it consistently, in about 2 weeks, you will find yourself becoming more aware of your thoughts and the way the different things affect your emotions and lure you towards certain activities. This will help you out a lot in becoming more conscious of your triggers.

Your next task is to do every task on your list cautiously so that you stay aware of it and the emotions it brings forth in you. Observe how different situations, experiences, people and thoughts make you feel and separate all those that make you think of shopping in one way or another. If you just picked up a magazine and saw an advertisement of a male model dressed in a crisp, gorgeous 3 piece and that makes you want to buy that for yourself, looking at adverts is your trigger. If you have a friend who is a hard-core shopaholic and being around her, makes you want to binge shop as well, she is the one who sets off your compulsive shopping behavior.

Observe yourself and the different triggers that activate your bad habit for a few days and note down all that information. Once you are quite well aware of how different activities and situations influence your buying behavior and the need to shop, move on to paying more attention to the rewards this behavior brings with itself because an understanding of the triggers, routine and rewards will better help you to pick out the right techniques to combat your problem.

Understand the Routine and Rewards

Pay attention to how you engage in shopping to understand your binge shopping routine as much as possible. This then helps in figuring out effective approaches to overcome the urge and soothe it. Focus on the following factors to understand the routine.

Do you only shop online?
Do you prefer visiting real stores and shopping from malls to making online purchases?
Do you like both online and offline shopping and engage in them as per your convenience?
How much time does it take you to decide on a purchase?
Do you always buy something impulsively or do you plan your shopping spree beforehand?

From thinking of what to buy to making the final purchase, how much time does it take you?

What are the different thoughts that run through your mind and emotions you experience while you are shopping?

How do you bring yourself to realize that you have shopped enough for the day and end the activity?

What thoughts and emotions do you experience when you end shopping? Do you feel sad or are you eager to have the package delivered to you in the case of online shopping or do you feel elated because you have bought something you like a lot?

Do you shop alone or with friends or other people and how does that affect your behavior?

Do you shop more when you are accompanied with people or do you shop less in that case?

Focus on all these questions and get answers to them to have an in depth comprehension of your shopping routine. Do write down everything as that helps you go through the written account and get better insight into your problem to address it effectively. Next, focus on the rewards this behavior brings along with itself so you know why you feel compelled to engage in it every now and then.

Know Your Rewards

Next or even in the meantime, observe your triggers and routine, pay attention to the different emotions and feelings that brew inside you after you have shopped for some things. Do you feel excited? Do you feel happy about buying something beautiful? Do you feel entertained while you shop and that is what is keeping you engaged in the act? Is shopping a means to fight off stress? Does shopping help you relax and has a therapeutic effect on you? Do you feel an urge to shop when you are with friends and hanging out in malls is your way to socialize with them?

Evaluate your feelings, pay attention to them and try to understand them so that you can know how you feel after you have shopped over and over again to better understand and realize the rewards associated with your compulsive shopping behavior.

You will be surprised to realize that the majority of the reasons why you shop and the benefits you derive out of the shopping experience aren't associated with your need to shop or buy something important, but are means to enjoy a certain feeling or get rid of a certain emotion.

Once you have more insight into your entire compulsive shopping behavior along with its triggers and rewards, you are now in a better place to understand your problem. Understand that no matter what triggered your addiction and in spite of the wonderful feelings you enjoy upon engaging in shopping, if it is interfering with your routine activities and disrupting the quality of life you would want, it is an unhealthy habit and needs to be changed. Shopping isn't bad because we do need some stuff in our life to live, but it is compulsive shopping that needs to be treated because that is what gets in the way of you living a meaningful life.

Tell yourself repeatedly that even though binge shopping does help you enjoy rewards, there are many healthier and more positive ways to enjoy the very same rewards and feel good without feeling guilty and wasting money in the process. Also, while your triggers do have quite some control over your thoughts right now and make you feel compelled to shop, you can control them so that nothing gets the better of you. Let us see how you can do that in the following chapter.

Chapter 5: Battling Your Triggers And Finding Healthier Alternatives To Shopping

Now that you have quite an in depth knowledge and awareness of what sets off your urge to shop incessantly, use that information to the best of your abilities to build an effective system that helps you keep your bad habit in check and slowly get better control on it. Here is how you can do that:

Manage Your Triggers

First, you need to learn to break off the first step that leads you towards a store, which means you need to train yourself to stop letting your triggers have control over you. Therefore, if you shop when you meet your brother because he has a chronic shopping addiction, maybe stop meeting him for a while until the time you gather better control of your addiction or schedule other fun activities that you can do together. If you experience the urge to shop every time you pick up a magazine, stop buying fashion magazines. If you are into home décor and cannot stop yourself from buying supplies and equipment to decorate your home more, stop going to IKEA every other day and shop elsewhere, where you will only have for instance, groceries if that is what you are buying.

It does take a lot of courage not to pay heed to a certain trigger especially if you have been doing it for a long time; however trust me, you can do that. You have it in you the ability to control yourself and keep your temptations in check and you can very well distract yourself from those temptations. To manage your triggers well, here are a few things you will have to try.

Set Incremental Goals: Often, you give in to your triggers after a few days of working on a goal mainly because it starts to drain your energy. A big goal is overwhelming and can exhaust you making it easier for you to surrender to your triggers. That can be avoided easily if you set incremental goals for yourself instead. Instead of focusing on breaking shopping addiction in 4 months, break down this goal into smaller, weekly milestones. Therefore, if for example you spend $500 on shopping every month, your 4 month goal could be divided into these milestones:

- Spend only $200 on shopping in week 1.
- Spend only $150 on shopping in week 2 and 3 each.
- Spend only $100 on shopping in week 4 and 5.
- Spend only $100 on shopping in week 6, 7 and 8.
- Spend only $80 on shopping in week 9, 10 and 11 each.
- Spend only $50 on shopping in week 12, 13 and 14.

- Spend less than $50 on shopping in week 15 and 16.

Remember this applies to purchasing needless stuff. There are things you need to buy such as groceries and other importance supplies in your home; so, this money excludes such expenditure.

Change Your Environment: Next, bring different positive changes to your environment that makes it conducive to success. If there are many magazines in your room related to the items you purchase the most, get rid of them. If you have pasted posters of fashion models in your room that makes you lean towards compulsive shopping, remove them. If your room or workplace is very dreary and messy, which triggers your depression leading you to shopping to feel better, get rid of the unnecessary clutter from it and make it brighter so that you do not feel dull and depressed when you enter it. Analyze your triggers and then assess your environment for any factors that contribute to the triggers and stimulate your addiction. Bring the necessary changes to your environment accordingly to slowly assuage your temptation to shop a lot and frequently.

Be Firm with Yourself and with Others: You need to slowly start being firmer and stricter with yourself first and then to all those around you who influence your compulsive shopping behavior in one way or another. Every time you wish to make a purchase or want to spend some time browsing an e-store, analyze your emotions and assess where that need is coming from. Ask yourself questions such as:

"Do I really need it?"

"On a scale of 1 to 10, how much do I need this product and why?"

"Do I have an alternative or a similar product that serves the same purpose?"

"What is my motive behind this purchase?"

"What do I lose if I don't make this purchase?"

"Will this purchase hurt my finances?" and similar questions to figure out whether you are buying out of desperation or actual need.

80 to 90% of the times, your answers will make you realize that you do not really need to make a certain purchase and it is your addiction trying to rule you. At that point, you need to be firm with yourself and instead of saying a direct No, distract yourself. Often, when we tell ourselves how we should not do something, we are quite likely to engage in that very practice after a while. If you tell yourself that you cannot eat that chocolate cake in your fridge, you are likely to find yourself sitting on the kitchen floor devouring the cake piece by piece after some time. This is human nature- we do what we are told not to. Thus, if you tell yourself how you must not make a certain purchase, you bet you will do exactly that. To keep that from happening, deal with yourself like a wise mother tackles a cranky kid.

Instead of saying a plain no, tell yourself how you have a few other things that serve the purpose and that you should rethink this purchase because what if an even better product comes along. Talk yourself out of the situation by thinking of how the money could be put to better use or how you should make a purchase tomorrow so you can buy more stuff.

Also, try distracting yourself by doing other tasks. You could get up and take a stroll in the park or drink water or watch something to distract your mind from shopping. As for being firm with others, distract them as well by saying things like how you are busy today or how it is better to shop over the weekend; and if need arises, firmly tell them how you are trying to have better control of your shopping and do not wish to engage in shopping right now. It will feel tough, but if you do it a few times, you will easily be able to convey your message loud and clear to all those who trigger your addiction.

Say No to Sales: Sales are one of the biggest reasons and factors that lure people into the compulsive shopping cycle. Be it end of season sales, Christmas sales, Black Friday sales or any other sales year around- they may seem as a great bargain, but in reality, they don't do you any good unless you really do want something which is an actual need.

Yes, things are available at great discounts on sales, but that's not true for every product or service. Often, there are products that aren't even worth $10, but they are marketed in a manner that makes you perceive them as a good bargain. In addition, even if something is a bargain, if you do not need it, then that is a waste of your money.

Therefore, make an effort to say NO to sales for good. Every year during the time of special sales, try not to watch too many commercials or videos. Install ad-blocking applications in your phone and laptop to block ads on all the websites you use. This way you won't be bombarded with ads and will manage your addiction.

Don't Visit Malls Unless Necessary: Try not to visit malls too often especially when you have a wallet full of money and feel a strong urge to spend the money on buying stuff. If possible, ask your accountability buddy to keep track of you so that he/ she makes sure you don't make any unnecessary trips to the mall and end up buying things for no good reason.

Stop Shopping your Emotions: Use meditation and mindfulness to be better aware of your emotions so that they do not pull you towards an e-store or that mall and make you engage in a meaningless purchase. Every time you feel emotional, engage in any other activity that can help you vent out your frustration and feel better. The next section discusses this better.

Have a Checklist: Whenever you go out shopping particularly grocery shopping, make a list of all the things you really need. Do not buy anything else that is not on the list. If you do forget to put something on the list, make do without it. This is a great hack to keep you from making unnecessary purchases because, when you go out without a list, you're likely to purchase whatever you find catchy which is quite likely to lead to compulsive buying and wastage of money.

As you keep track of your triggers and slowly learn to manage them effectively, find different activities that you can engage in to take your mind off the stressful situations you are going through in life. This helps you enjoy more or less the same rewards binge shopping provided you with making it easier to manage your addiction.

Look for Substitutes to Enjoy Same Rewards

There are many healthy ways to ward off stress, anxiety and depression and have better control of your nerves so you don't give in to your temptation every time it strikes you. Whether you are bored or exhausted or hurt or jealous or going through any emotion that you don't like and want to get rid of, there are other activities that help you enjoy the same results. Here are some good ideas for you.

Paint or Do Something Crafty: Every time you feel a huge wave of stress completely take over you, wash it away by engaging in an arts and crafts related activity. Make pots, paint, draw, create jewelry or do anything creative you enjoy, to take your mind off the stressful experience and stay away from online and offline stores. If you enjoy coloring, get stress releasing coloring books for adults and color away every time you feel a strong urge to shop because you feel overwhelmed or anxious.

Dance off Your Stress: Dancing is a great way to release negativity and lower cortisol levels. Cortisol is a hormone associated with stress and when its levels in your body increase, you are likely to feel frustrated and resort to your addiction to feel better. To get rid of it, dance like nobody is watching you to your favorite upbeat song and you will surely feel much better and relaxed than before.

Read Good Books: Get your hands on a nice book of your favorite genre and pick it up every time you feel your hands moving towards your laptop opening your favorite online store.

Go for Walks: Ensure that you go out for a nice stroll in the park every time you feel bored or stressed. Fresh air relaxes you and takes your mind off the addiction.

Talk to Good Friends: Build a support system around you composing of supportive and understanding loved ones who are aware of your problem and want to help you get rid of it. Talk to any one of them every time you feel swamped by negativity and want to shop your heart out. You can create a group comprising of all these people on Whatsapp and keep everyone posted of you shopping related activities so they can encourage you to work on your milestones.

Connect with people going through the Same Problem: Facebook groups have emerged as a completely new world of possibilities and positivity. Make use of that by creating a support group for all those who are trying to break free of their shopping addiction and share your journey with them. You are likely to inspire others and be inspired by other people's stories to stay true to your commitment. Together, all of you can emerge as winners in the end and completely break your addiction.

Experiment with these activities and any other positive activity that provides you the same rewards as shopping did and engage in it every time you feel an urge to buy more stuff to slowly let go of your addiction.

Conclusion

We have come to the end of the book. Thank you for reading and congratulations for reading until the end. Always remember that you are a strong warrior well able to overcome your addiction and live a fulfilling and happier life free from your need to Shop all the time.

Finally, if you found the book valuable, can you recommend it to others? One way to do that is to post a review on Amazon.

Printed in Great Britain
by Amazon